A Healthier You!

A HEALTHIER YOU!

ALSO BY SPENCER COFFMAN

A Guide To Deception
Relax And Unwind
Work Less Live More

A HEALTHIER YOU!

A HEALTHIER YOU!

101 Powerful Tips For A Fitter, Healthier You!

BY
SPENCER COFFMAN

A HEALTHIER YOU!

While every precaution has been taken in the preparation of this book, the author and/or publisher assumes no responsibility for errors or omissions, or for damages resulting from the use of the information contained herein.

A HEALTHIER YOU 101 POWERFUL TIPS FOR A FITTER, HEALTHIER YOU

First edition. May 2016.

ISBN: 978-15466180-9-6 (Paperback)
ISBN: 978-1-5337396-5-0 (Digital)
ISBN: 978-1-0942259-2-0 (Audio)

Written by Spencer Coffman.
SpencerCoffman.com

"Discover Simple Techniques To Becoming Fit And Healthy And Staying That Way, Starting Today!"

This Guide Will Show You Easy Ways To Become A Healthier You -- No Fluff, No Fillers... Only Useful Techniques You Can Start Using Today

From: Spencer Coffman

Dear Friend,

Are you looking to **get fit?**
Is it about time you **get in shape?**
Do you want to **eat well and healthy?**
Do you find it a **struggle** to do it all with your busy routine?
If you do, read on, because I'm about to share something very special with you...

It's Not Your Fault!

With all the misleading information out there, **yo-yo diets,** weight loss pills, and scams, you don't know who or where to turn to.

It's not your fault. If you've been caught up in any

of these **vicious cycles,** it's time to relax because I'm about to present to you **simple techniques** to help you get fit and healthy.

These techniques have **nothing** to do with yo-yo diets. These are **essential** health and fitness tips you should know. From changing your mindset to the things you eat. It really does start in the mind.

You could have the latest and greatest weight loss or fitness program out there, but if your mind is not prepared for it all, then you're wasting your time and money.

So without further ado...

Introducing:
A Healthier You!

A valuable guide sharing 101 powerful tips on health, fitness, weight control, cardio health, and working out.

EXACTLY WHAT'S INSIDE THIS GUIDE?

101 powerful tips on health and fitness. Easy to read. Easy to implement. Straight to the point.

The **most important rule** to getting fit and healthy. Don't miss this tip!

Why you should **never skip breakfast.** Believe it or not, you'll actually lose weight by eating breakfast.

How to use the power of relaxation to your advantage.

Don't avoid carbs. People will tell you to avoid carbs, but did you know there are good and bad carbs? This tip will explain.

How eating 5 to 6 meals a day will **assist** you in your weight control program.

How to control your cravings so you don't end up eating unhealthy foods and drinks. This technique will show you how to stop those temptations.

How to maintain a **positive attitude** regardless of the situation you're in. This is a very important step to achieving your goals.

Relaxation by meditating and breathing.

How stretching relaxes your mind, body, and spirit.

And Much, much more!

Get Instant Access To This Package Right Now!

A HEALTHIER YOU!

It's a steal of a deal!

So go ahead. You have nothing to lose. Grab your copy today!

"Yes! I'm tired of feeling unhealthy and I really want to start experiencing better health and fitness today.

So please send me my copy of "A Healthier You" - so I can learn how to get my health in order right away!

Claim Your Copy Today!

A Healthier You!

A HEALTHIER YOU!

Table of Contents

Introduction

1	Stay hydrated.
2	Your mom was right, never skip breakfast.
3	Take fish oil supplements.
4	Work up a sweat.
5	Add variety to your exercise routine.
6	Get enough sleep.
7	Enjoy mind and body exercises.
8	Learn relaxation techniques.
9	Ditch the chips for healthier snack options.
10	Discover the healthy goodness of green tea.
11	Take vitamin supplements.
12	Wash your hands often.
13	Get rid of unhealthy vices.
14	Take annual health tests.
15	Be kind to yourself.
16	Stay motivated.
17	Drink alcohol in moderation.
18	Limit sugar in your diet as much as possible.
19	Eat complex carbohydrates.
20	Cut down your caffeine.
21	Push yourself.
22	Take it from Nike, JUST DO IT.
23	Watch what you put in your grocery cart.
24	Eat 5 to 6 meals a day.
25	Eat at home.

A HEALTHIER YOU!

26 Incorporate physical activities in your daily life.
27 Be selective on the shows you watch on TV.
28 Make smart food choices.
29 Maintain at least one hobby.
30 Bask in love.
31 Go organic.
32 Avoid negative people and situations.
33 Explore.
34 Don't confuse thirst with hunger.
35 Eat at a leisurely pace.
36 Avoid stress eating.
37 Avoid eating while watching TV or going to the movies.
38 Teach yourself to control cravings.
39 Get support from family and friends.
40 Beat temptations through distraction.
41 Keep a diary or journal.
42 Don't overlook the importance of emotional fitness.
43 Don't indulge too much on one thing.
44 Find a fitness buddy.
45 Ride a bike to work.
46 Be conscious with your food portions.
47 Increase fiber in your daily diet.
48 Enjoy after dinner walks.
49 Bake, steam, or grill instead of frying.
50 Avoid eating at all you can eat buffets.
51 Only take enough food you can eat.
52 Start your meals with salads.
53 Replace sugar with honey.
54 Avoid skipping meals.
55 Trade baked goods with fresh fruits.
56 When eating out, choose the healthiest meals.
57 Avoid using condiments.

Table of Contents

58   When traveling, check out gym facilities.

59   Do your research on local restaurants that offer healthy alternatives.

60   Bring your lunch.

61   Trade your recliner with an exercise ball.

62   Use your break time wisely.

63   Conduct a meeting on the go.

64   Invest in a pedometer.

65   Learn to modify.

66   Take vacations from work, not from good health.

67   Learn to express your feelings.

68   Maintain a positive attitude.

69   Try meditation.

70   Reinforce your faith.

71   Stay young at heart.

72   Stay in touch with friends.

73   Perform regular stretching exercises.

74   Keep talking.

75   Stop smoking.

76   Aim high.

77   Keep yourself updated.

78   Know your body.

79   Grill it up.

80   Treat your brain like any other muscle.

81   Get nutty.

82   Stay protected.

83   Mind your posture.

84   Avoid processed food products.

85   Always carry a water bottle wherever you go.

86   Get plenty of fresh air.

87   Take advantage of natural sunlight.

88   Take the stairs.

89   For women, visit gynecologist regularly.

90   Walk and stretch during road travel.

91   Visit your dentist regularly.

92   Workout with kids.

93   Substitute emails for walks.

94   Warm up before exercise.

95   Take a stand.

96   Park farther.

97   Use chicken breast and take off the skin.

98   Learn to decipher food labels.

99   Just chew it.

100   Always choose to plan ahead.

101   Keep moving forward.

Conclusion

Appendix A: Checklist

Appendix B: Resource Cheat Sheet

Appendix C: Mind Map

Introduction

Fact:

*If you want more out of life,
you need to be ready to commit,
and invest more into staying fit
and eating right. ~ Spencer Coffman*

There are an insurmountable amount of diet plans and exercise programs that have all been sprouting like mushrooms over the past few years. That is probably something that will never change. People always want to get in shape and have a great looking body. The bad thing is that all of these programs claim to provide the fastest results. The good thing is that all of these programs have the same basic principles, which are diet and exercise. That's it, the basic equation to staying fit and healthy is having a proper diet and getting regular exercise.

It has been called by many names, defined in so many ways, and presented in so many forms. However, the bottom line is that all health and fitness programs boil down to these two fundamentals: DIET and EXERCISE. There is no other way to go about it, especially if you want lasting results.

Yet, despite this common knowledge on what needs

to be done to stay fit and healthy, most people still struggle to maintain that slim and sexy look. More and more everyday, people are going in the opposite direction. This country is gaining weight exponentially, yet millions of people say they wish they could be thinner and more fit!

As a result, the weight loss industry has become a highly lucrative market. Food manufacturers, nutrition experts, gyms, plastic surgeons, and more, feed on the growing desperation, and depression, of overweight and obese individuals.

Even though the equation to fitness and health is so simple and straightforward, it remains a great challenge. Basically, it is easier said than done. With the demands of daily living, work-related stresses, social pressures, life changes, holidays, travels, winter seasons, and everything else in between; it is a great difficulty to stay in shape. There are simply too many easy, fast, convenient, great tasting foods out there! All of which are contributing factors that can disrupt fitness routines and upset diet regimens.

The real challenge here is how you can possibly stay resolute and consistent with the program, despite internal and external factors that often come into play.

This book is designed to help you equip yourself with tips, tricks, and practical advice on how you can stay fit and healthy in the modern times. That way you can have everything you need to become a fitter, healthier you!

Introduction

It doesn't have to be a constant struggle. Fitness and healthy living is not a temporary phase or a convenient solution that you can readily pull out from your closet in time for the summer season or during special occasions. If you want lasting results, ditch the two-week plan or the six-month program. Make health and fitness an integral part of your lifestyle, as it should be. You need to break the habit of always eating junk food and get into the habit of making your own healthy food. It isn't easy, but it will get easier as you start to break the cravings for those "bad for you" foods.

Read on and find out you can live, breathe, eat, move, and think healthy!

A HEALTHIER YOU!

101 Powerful Tips For A Fitter, Healthier You!

1   Stay hydrated.

This is one of the most important pieces of advice that you can ever get when it comes to staying fit and healthy. Drinking water every chance you get, or at least every couple of hours, will make your body so much healthier. Water helps ensure your body systems will keep running smoothly. Water flushes your system and helps remove toxins. It also plays a vital role in weight loss and provides you with energy. So don't forget to drink up!

2   Your mom was right, never skip breakfast.

You have probably heard it over and over how breakfast is the most important meal of the day. And it really is. A lot of people seem to think skipping breakfast will help them lose weight faster. This could not be further than the truth! Think about it, you go all night without eating. That is eight hours. Your body needs nourishment. The first thing that you should do when you wake up is to drink at least sixteen ounces of water. Then you should make yourself a nice high protein breakfast. You have already gone eight hours without food; if you skip breakfast, you turn eight hours into twelve or fourteen hours. That is not healthy and will cause your body to go into conservation mode. That means it will begin to store fat cells, thus causing you to gain weight!

According to numerous medical studies, people who skip breakfast have increased risks of gaining weight. Breakfast helps stabilize the body's metabolism. Ditching your first meal of the day will result in an increase in LDL levels, or bad cholesterol, and lower insulin levels. The increase in bad cholesterol in the body will result to clogged arteries, which can lead to a number of serious health complications such as heart disease. There is also that little known fact that people tend to take in higher calories all throughout the day after missing their breakfast. If you are trying to lose weight, have an all protein breakfast so that it keeps you full throughout the day.

3 Take fish oil supplements.

Recent studies conducted by the University of Western Ontario revealed that regular intake of fish oil supplements can speed up the burning of calories by as much as 400 more calories. Fish oil supplements are rich in Omega 3, which is also effective in the prevention of the hardening of the arteries, which is one of the leading causes of heart disease. Fish oil, and other essential fatty acids, or EFA's, are also excellent for your brain. They can help prevent the risk of dementia and Alzheimer's.

When taking fish oil supplements, make sure that you are getting a good supplement. Often times, the generic brands may have mercury in them. Or they may have a diluted dose. When getting fish oil, you need to do your research. It would also be a great idea to consult a natural or homeopathic doctor.

4   Work up a sweat.

Make exercise a part of your daily routine. Regular exercise helps keep the heart healthy. It also will provide you with more energy throughout the day. If you do a high-intensity workout for a half hour in the morning, then your body will continue to burn calories at a high rate for up to six hours after that!

There are a number of ways that you can incorporate exercise into your lifestyle. It's simply a matter of finding one that is best for you. Try to exercise at least three to four times a week. That way you will begin to make it a habit. You don't have to do much. In fact, you will be surprised how many calories a simple jog or brisk walk can burn. To give you an idea, here are a few examples:

Biking at a leisurely pace for 1 hour -- a total of 230 to 340 calories burned

Walking at a moderate pace for 1 hour – a total of 205 to 300 calories burned

Mowing the lawn for 1 hour – a total of 300 to 450

calories burned

Jogging at a moderate pace for 1 hour -- a total of 300 to 600 calories burned

High-intensity workout for 1 hour -- a total of 800 to 1200 calories burned

5   Add variety to your exercise routine.

Keep things light and fun by changing your fitness routine every now and then. Explore activities that aid weight loss, go outside, and jog along the park or by the beach. Consider taking up strength training, mountain climbing, cycling, and other fun activities that can make exercise more fun and exciting. It may also be a good idea to find some free workout classes at your local gyms or universities. Then attend a few different sessions each week.

If you are not the type of person to go outside and run around like some sort of fitness maniac, then you can work out at home! Simply purchase some DVD's and do a different one every day. The key is you need to do them! If you don't work out you won't have any results. Do whatever you have to do. Simply make sure that you are doing, instead of not doing.

6   Get enough sleep.

With the fast-paced lifestyle and grueling schedules, sleep is often taken for granted. The average person needs to have at least seven to eight hours of sleep every night. If you want to maintain a healthy weight, sleep should be given equal importance. The time when you are asleep is the only time the body can heal and repair itself. Therefore, you need to make sure that you are allowing your body to recharge. Think about it, if you use your cell phone for eight hours a day, do you plug it in at night? Of course! You need to recharge your phone. Your body is similar, in that after being in use for sixteen hours, it needs to rest and recharge. Your body needs sleep so that it can heal and repair. Lack of sleep causes so many ailments and impairs brain function, so make sure you get enough ZZZ's.

7   Enjoy mind and body exercises.

Consider taking yoga or tai chi classes. They specialize in focusing your mind on only one task at a time, and are very relaxing. This will help you to let go of stress and create a much healthier body. These exercises not only stretch your muscles and strengthen the bones, sinews, and joints, they can also help you relax mentally. Of course, you have to be willing to relax your mind in order for your mind to really relax.

Mind and body exercises are a great way to wind down after a long and grueling day at work. They can help ease pain and anxiety as well as speed up recovery time. They are an excellent way to burn calories without the high-intensity workout. If you are conducting extensive workouts a few times a week, then it is extremely important that you substitute a few of these low-intensity relaxation workouts in between the high-intensity workouts. They will help repair your muscles and relax your joints. The best part is, that you are still burning calories!

8   Learn relaxation techniques.

It's no secret that stress can contribute to weight gain and the development of chronic diseases. By learning relaxation responses, you can stop the adverse effects that come with stress. Several of the popular relaxation techniques include breathing exercises, journaling, visualization, and laughter, among others. If you deal with a serious amount of stress on a daily basis, teach your body how to best cope with it.

One of the best ways to deal with stress is to work out. This channels your stress into something that will also help you to get fit. If you have a rough day, hit the gym hard and really push yourself in the weights. Tear down your muscles so that you can really feel the burn. Then take a nice relaxing shower and have a healthy smoothie afterward. You'll be surprised how relaxed and refreshed you feel.

9   Ditch the chips for healthier snack options.

Cultivate smarter food choices to stay fit and healthy. This includes choosing your snacks with more thought and consideration. If you enjoy a bag of chips while watching TV, or movie, replace it with healthier snack choices. There are many healthier options that will also satisfy that craving to eat something crunchy. The best option is probably a cucumber. Eat it straight from the refrigerator. They are very high in B vitamins and will help provide you with energy. Another great choice would be celery and peanut butter. That will give you a whole lot of crunchiness and some protein as well. Of course, you could also eat an apple with your peanut butter. But be careful, fruit is metabolized as sugar, which converts into fat in your body.

Keep your healthy snacks readily on hand so you won't be tempted to indulge in junk food. Spend a few hours one evening a week to cut up and prepare all of your vegetables. Place them in Ziplocs so that they will be ready for you to take to work or grab when you need a snack. If you make your healthy food convenient and easily accessible, then it will help ensure that you eat that when you are hungry instead of reaching for the bag of chips. In addition, make sure you don't have junk food and unhealthy food products in your desk and pantry. By keeping it out of sight, you won't feel deprived.

10 Discover the healthy goodness of green tea.

Take it from the Japanese who have been skinny for centuries, and discover how green tea can aid in rapid weight loss. Green tea has numerous health benefits. It provides the body with caffeine, which is excellent after a workout. It also satisfies your thirst for something other than water. You can drink it hot, like coffee, or cold like soda and other fizzy drinks. It is a great alternative to sugary drink choices.

In addition to being great for weight loss and calorie burning, green tea has been known to work well with a number of health conditions including: rheumatoid arthritis, cardiovascular diseases, impaired immune function, infections, high cholesterol levels, and even certain forms of cancer. Therefore, get out and buy some green tea today!

As always, make sure that the bags you purchase have good whole ingredients. Preservatives and fillers won't help you. So buy bags and brew it yourself. If you need it sweetened, then add a little honey or stevia. Nothing else, other sugars can be metabolized too rapidly and stored as fat cells.

11 Take vitamin supplements.

If you are trying to cut down on your calorie intake, chances are you may also be compromising your nutrition. After all, it is hard to eat all the time when you are trying to lose weight. You will eat more if you work out. That is a simple fact. You are burning more calories, and therefore, need more nutrients. So make sure that you are eating more of the right foods. It is also a great idea to add some supplements into your diet because you are burning so many nutrients in your workout that you don't normally burn.

The best way to augment the depleted vitamins and minerals in the body is through vitamins. Find a great multi-vitamin that you can take once a day. When choosing supplements, stay away from the mass marketed brands at popular stores like Target, Wal-Mart, CVS, and Walgreens. You need to go to a real nutrition company and get some quality products. Talk to a naturopath or homeopathic doctor and see what they recommend. Chances are, you can find an amazing multi-vitamin for around $30 a month.

12   Wash your hands often.

An excellent way to avoid getting sick and to stay healthy is to wash your hands thoroughly and regularly. This is a very basic habit that has probably been ingrained in you since early childhood. However, it is often forgotten about and overlooked. Below are some guidelines on when you should wash your hands. Of course, there are many more instances in which you should wash your hands. However, this will get you started.

Always wash your hands before:

- Preparing meals
- Eating
- Treating wounds
- Giving medication
- Caring for the injured and sick

Always wash your hands after:

- Handling food, especially when handling raw meat and poultry
- Using the toilet

- Changing diapers
- Touching toys, pets, and trash
- Coughing, blowing of nose, and sneezing into hands
- Treating wounds
- Caring for the injured and sick
- Handling chemicals, garbage or anything contaminated

13   Get rid of unhealthy vices.

In order to truly become a healthier you, you need to work hard to cultivate healthy habits and ditch those that pose adverse effects on your health. Habits like smoking, drinking heavily, watching too much TV, disorganization, stress, et cetera are all detrimental to your health and wellbeing. In addition, anything in excess can be bad for you and you don't want your health to suffer the consequences. Therefore, do everything in moderation.

Having a few drinks a week is okay. Some are even good for you. Smoking is pretty much always bad. However, one here and there could help with stress. If you drink soda, only drink one once in a while. Everything in moderation, and try to completely eliminate those things that are always going to be bad for you, like smoking and soda.

14   Take annual health tests.

Annual physical examinations are generally covered by health insurance. If you have that option, then take advantage of it, even if you don't like doctors. You are already paying an insurance premium, go in and get something for the money you are giving them. If it isn't covered by your insurance, then find a cheap clinic. Often times there are free clinics or universities that offer specials and discounted prices. Routine tests are important to detect health problems at an early stage before they grow into a serious health issue. You could also go to a homeopathic doctor or naturopath, as often times they can fix problems that medical doctors will merely treat instead of fix.

15   Be kind to yourself.

This one is twofold. You must be kind to yourself like you would to other people. Don't be too hard on yourself. There are plenty of other people out in the world that will insult you and tell you that you are no good. DON'T do it to yourself. You need to always have a positive attitude. Don't be whiney and pouty when something goes wrong. Persevere and be great. You can do it. You simply have to want to.

The second part is that you need to treat yourself every now and then. This has to be once in a while. Monthly is an excellent time frame. It can be something incredibly simple like getting an ice-cream cone when you notice your favorite flavor of the day, or something like enjoying a great meal out. Other activities may include pampering, such as getting your hair done at a posh salon, or scheduling a massage appointment. Basically, it can be anything that you enjoy doing that will allow you to break away from the demands and pressures of daily living. It is something that will help you to slow down, recharge, and truly appreciate the activity.

16   Stay motivated.

It can be difficult to stay on track with a health and fitness program if you are no longer motivated. Seek inspiration, and find ways to stay motivated to make smarter choices and right decisions every single day. You are constantly faced with choices that pose real temptations, such as choosing between watching TV and working out, or choosing between a chocolate chip cookie and a vegetable snack. Motivation will help you make the right decision.

If you have a desire and a goal in mind, then you can be motivated to reach that goal. Therefore, if you start to lose motivation, set some new goals and promise yourself some rewards when you achieve them. That way you will be motivated to achieve the reward, which will help you fulfill the goal and make the right choices in order to achieve that goal. Essentially, it is a reverse snowball effect.

17   Drink alcohol in moderation.

Alcohol shows up in almost every social event, especially during the holiday season. Learn to limit your intake to no more than one or two drinks, since too much alcohol can disrupt your sleep and make you feel sluggish the following day, not to mention contribute to extra calories. However, keep in mind that some forms of alcohol are better for you than others. Any sugary drinks are obviously bad for you, so is beer because it contains carbs. Basically, the only alcoholic drinks that can be healthy are red wine and hard liquor. Of course, these must be consumed in moderation in order to have health benefits.

18   Limit sugar in your diet as much as possible.

We all know how sugar can be detrimental to your health. The problem is that it is in so many products. Therefore, make sure to read the labels and learn to steer clear of any processed food products because they are most likely laden with too much sugar. Nutrition experts recommend limiting added sugar to no more than ten tablespoons a day. Of course, it would be best if you ate no sugar at all, but sometimes it cannot be avoided.

Sugar can come in so many forms and under many names. You need to be vigilant and always read the labels of foods before you eat them. In general, you need to steer clear of any foods that contain high amounts of the ingredients that are listed below.

- Glucose
- High fructose corn syrup
- Lactose
- Honey
- Fruit juice concentrates
- Molasses
- Maltose

- Sucrose
- Brown sugar
- Fructose

To give you an idea of the sugar content on some of the popular food products and beverages, refer to the following data:

Regular soda	33%
Candies	16%
Cakes, pies, and cookies	13%
Fruit drinks	10%

Individuals who are constantly exposed to consumption of food products with high sugar content also increase their calorie intake and lower micronutrient supply. In addition, they are more prone to the development of diabetes than those who don't eat sugar. The bottom line is that you need to limit your sugar. The less sugar, the better off you'll be.

19   Eat complex carbohydrates.

When it comes to losing weight and eating right, we all know we need to watch our carb intake. Some people say that there are good carb sources that are perfectly safe to eat such as whole grains. In addition, the FDA recommends 55% of daily calorie supply should be derived from carbohydrates. However, you need to closely monitor the sources of your carbohydrates, as there is a huge difference between complex and simple carbohydrates. Basically, if you want to be healthy, try not to eat carbs. It is as simple as that.

Limit yourself to three to five carbs a day. A potato, a serving of corn, a slice of bread, a half-cup of oats, and a beer, are all examples of one serving of carbs.

Simple carbohydrates are normally found in pasta, rice, potatoes, chips, bread, sweets, et cetera. They contain high amounts of sugar that need to be broken down by the body. In fact, two slices of bread are metabolized into the same sugar as a twelve-ounce can of soda. This type of sugar will be quickly burned, and provide you with a burst of energy. However, it will be followed by a crash that begins when your body starts to convert all of the sugar into fat cells. This is the reason why many diets restrict the intake of carbohydrate-rich food. Simple carbohydrates can contribute to weight gain and are especially risky for pregnant women.

On the other hand, complex carbohydrates, while containing sugar also feature more complex chains, making it more difficult to break it down. Therefore, they are absorbed and used more slowly, which allows the body plenty of time to regulate the absorption of the ingredients. Another great benefit of complex carbs is the high fiber content, which adds bulk to the diet, effectively warding of hunger at the same time alleviating and preventing constipation. Examples of complex carbs include foods like steel cut oats, brown long grain rice, whole flours such as spelt and sorghum, and some whole grain breads that are usually seedy and very dense, like Ezekiel bread.

20   Cut down your caffeine.

Too much caffeine can be bad for your health. Limit your intake to one to four servings per day. Perhaps you have two cups of coffee in the morning and a cup of tea in the afternoon. Whatever your designation, make sure you know how much you are consuming. Use common sense; a standard coffee mug should be about eight ounces. The truth is that a lot of people are silent victims of caffeine addiction with common symptoms that include irritability, anxiety, upset stomach, poor concentration, insomnia, and depression, among others.

Caffeine has become a lifetime drug addiction for many. In essence, it is a toxic substance that should always be taken in moderation. Like sugar, it has the tendency to overstimulate, and then weaken, the adrenal glands. Weak adrenals result in fatigue because they are responsible for fighting stress. When they become overworked, they begin to shut down, which is a bad thing.

If you are not really hooked into drinking coffee, avoid the addiction at all cost. Like illegal drugs, caffeine also has its own host of unpleasant symptoms during withdrawal. Remember, everything in moderation.

21   Push yourself.

You are the only person who knows what you are capable of. You need to always be ready and willing to push yourself to the limit and beyond. This doesn't mean being hard on yourself. There is a huge difference between being hard on yourself and adhering to self-discipline. You need to have self-discipline, and lots of it. That way you will be able to continue working hard to achieve your goals and become a healthier you.

Push yourself in a positive way but don't allow self-imposed pressure to overwhelm you. Instead, allow pressure to motivate you. Work harder to get tasks done and then relax when they are complete. That way you will train yourself to accomplish something and reap the reward of relaxation.

22   Take it from Nike, JUST DO IT.

Most people's best skill is procrastination. Many people are willing victims of procrastination and always put off exercise and diet for another day. It seems that it has become a national pastime to simply do something later. Don't fall into this mentality! If you already are a procrastinator, then you need to break that habit right now!

Instead of overthinking and overplanning things, simply go ahead and do them. When you see a task, start it and work until you finish it. You must learn to see things all the way through to the end. You will soon find that your motivation will be greatly increased. In addition, you will discover that the hardest part of any task is getting started.

23 Watch what you put in your grocery cart.

One cardinal rule that you need to vigilantly follow is to never do your grocery shopping on an empty stomach. If you have to go shopping and are hungry, then eat something before you go into the store. Otherwise, you will find yourself falling prey to compulsive buying. As you walk through the isles, you will buy anything and everything that looks good. Then you will get to the register to find a huge bill waiting for you and a cart full of junk food that you shouldn't be taking home. Therefore, it is essential to prepare a list of things you need and to make sure to stick to that list. When making your list, make sure to stick to whole, fresh food, products and high protein foods.

24 Eat 5 to 6 meals a day.

Many people who go on a diet often complain about dealing with hunger pangs and that sense of deprivation. That is because people on a diet make the mistake of thinking that they are restricted to eating only a few times a day. This is a terrible way to diet, especially when you are combining diet with exercise.

The best way to combat these feelings of deprivation is to replace your three large meals with five or six small meals. This will prevent you from overeating and caving into temptation. In addition, regular food intake can pump up your metabolism, which will burn more calories. Therefore, eat throughout the entire day, and make sure that you are eating healthy foods.

25 Eat at home.

One major contributing factor to weight gain is the propensity to eat fast food meals, takeout, and microwave dinners. All of which are heavily laden with calories. Another problem is that they are very high in saturated fats and sodium. These foods are terrible for your organs, contribute to rapid weight gain, and are instantly stored as fat cells within your body. Therefore, try your best to avoid eating them.

Of course, it will require extra effort to prepare meals from scratch, but it's worth it because you should never compromise your health with convenience. If you are short of time during the week and convenience meals are an important part of your life, then create your own fast food meals. Spend a few hours a week preparing several meals in advance. Then take some of those leftovers and package them up in containers to place in the freezer. That way, when you are in a hurry, you can simply pop them into the microwave for a healthy fast food meal.

26 Incorporate physical activities in your daily life.

Maximize every chance you get to move your body and work out. You don't really need to go to the gym to burn calories, there are so many ways you can pump up your metabolism by making simple changes, such as taking the stairs instead of the elevator, or parking further away so you will be forced walk. Play with your kids, or perform push-ups during commercial breaks. Do everything you can to stay active throughout the entire day. This will not only burn calories, but will also make you feel better. This is because you will increase your metabolism and blood flow, thereby increasing your energy and self-satisfaction.

27 Be selective on the shows you watch on TV.

The whole concept is to limit TV time before you unwittingly turn into a couch potato. If you tend to enjoy watching TV too much and too often, you won't realize how much time you spend in front of the tube. Therefore, you need to make sure to limit your TV time. Instead of spending several hours watching one show after the next, make the choice to watch two shows each night. This way it will be something to which you look forward.

According to studies, too much TV can lead to early death. A sedentary lifestyle can take off years from your life and increase the risk of heart disease. While TV in itself is not harmful, unless you are practicing some of the stupidity portrayed in most of today's modern TV entertainment, being stationary is. Constantly sitting in the same position for hours leads to the general absence of muscle movement. Habitually not moving for extended periods of time significantly disrupts the body's metabolism. Therefore, limit your TV time.

28   Make smart food choices.

Some diets impose impossible restrictions that are simply not practical or sustainable. The goal is not to simply go on a diet for a few weeks and lose weight in time for summer. It isn't to work out extra hard every day so that you can go home and eat whatever you want either. The goal here is for you to start making choices that will become a part of your lifestyle. You need to make healthy living your new way of life. Sure, you can eat some junk food now and then, but you need to make sure to do so in moderation. The majority of the foods you buy, and consume, need to be healthy whole foods. Make it your way of life, and pretty soon it will be so natural that you won't even like some of the junk foods you used to eat.

29   Maintain at least one hobby.

Find an activity that you are passionate about and that you won't mind doing for hours. You need to learn to enjoy something that isn't work related. Something that you only do for the simple reason that it is fun for you to do so. Other people may see it as a waste of time, but that's okay. As long as you enjoy it, and it is somewhat constructive and active, then it is perfect. May it be photography, visiting museums, attending sales and auctions, or spending hours in a bookstore. Pursue the things that bring the greatest joy to you.

Having an enjoyable hobby is great for your mental wellbeing. It is something that will occupy your time and relieve some of the stress and anxiety from your day-to-day life. You must find something that you love doing so that you become completely engaged in it. While you are performing your hobby, you need to put everything else out of your mind and focus purely on enjoying the moment.

30   Bask in love.

Whether you have a significant other, family, friends, or even your pet dog, take the time to connect with them and enjoy their company. Companionship is something that is instilled in the human DNA. It is something that everyone longs for and needs. Even the castaway had Wilson, his volleyball. Having a good friend makes life so much easier to go through. So don't be afraid to put yourself out there and make some friends. Bask in the love that surrounds you and learn to recognize the signs of love that people show you. It isn't all about romantic love. Someone who does a favor for you out of the goodness of their heart is showing you their love. Therefore, work to establish connections and nurture relationships. It can do wonders for your health and wellbeing.

31   Go organic.

You have probably heard reports on how even fresh produce today is exposed to chemicals and pesticides. Well, it is, and even though it is healthier for you than processed foods, you are still being exposed to some nasty chemicals. Therefore, it is generally best to get your food from organic sources. The bad thing is that organic food is much more expensive than regular food. The good thing is that with the growing demand for such products, you can easily find different varieties and brands that are labeled organically grown or produced.

A cheaper alternative would be for you to grow some of your own food. If you can make it work, this is an excellent option. Growing your own food provides a satisfaction that cannot be explained. However, if it isn't an option, then try to find organic food when it goes on sale. If all else fails, remember there is no price tag for good health, right?

32   Avoid negative people and situations.

Too much emotional stress can wreak havoc to your wellbeing. This does not mean you should avoid confrontations altogether, but learn when and where to draw the lines. There is no use being around people who belittle you and undermine your dreams and goals. Leave them for the birds. You need to be around people that are like-minded to you. Associate with people who will support and encourage you.

When you come across people who are full of themselves and only care about themselves, then go the other way. You must limit your exposure to people that stress you out and are negative. Prolonged exposure to stress can trigger binge eating and depression, which will ultimately lead to weight gain and mental instability. Therefore, associate with people who you enjoy being around, not those who are taxing and exhausting.

33   Explore.

Exploring doesn't always mean traveling and seeing the world. However, if you have the means and opportunity then, by all means, do so. If you don't, then seek to explore the world that is all around you. How many places are in the city in which you live? Hundreds, thousands, have you been to them all? Move beyond your comfort zone every once in a while and make an effort to go to some of those places. Take the time and do it. It will be worth it. Don't be afraid to get lost doing so. After all, getting lost is something that all explorers experience.

The practice of adding something new, and pursuing something worthwhile, will help keep you active and alive. It breaks the usual humdrum of everyday life and opens up your world to vast horizons. In addition, think of all the experience and knowledge you will gain. Therefore, be open to new experiences, and be more accommodating to change. New experiences will lead to deeper self-discovery and a more meaningful life.

34   Don't confuse thirst with hunger.

The human body has difficulty differentiating thirst from hunger. Your brain simply tells you that you need something. Therefore, when you begin to believe you are hungry, start drinking some water. Avoid indulging in food right away and only drink water. Then, after ten or fifteen minutes, if you still feel hungry, go ahead and eat. Often times, the water will fill you up and take away your hunger. If it didn't, then you will still eat less as a result of the water that is now in your stomach. It is always a good practice to begin every meal with a glass of water. Doing so will help you prevent overeating.

35 Eat at a leisurely pace.

Enjoy your food, and chew it thoroughly. It will usually take twenty minutes before you feel full, so it's important not to gorge down your food. A number of studies have confirmed that people who tend to eat slowly consume a lesser amount of calories, enough to help you lose as much as twenty pounds per year. The brain takes time to register fullness of stomach, which means that by eating slowly, you have more time to realize that you are already full.

Make an effort to take up the practice of eating until you feel like you are about three quarters full. Don't worry, you will soon feel full when the rest of your food makes it into your stomach. If you eat until you are completely full then you are actually overeating. This is because your body senses the food after it makes it part way down your esophagus. If you eat until you are completely full then you still have an esophagus full of food that is not yet being sensed by your body. This is why sometimes you feel over full a half hour after eating.

36   Avoid stress eating.

Unfortunately, many people become unwitting victims to this pitfall. If you feel the need to binge eat to relieve stress, ask yourself what triggered it. Take the time to figure it out so that you will know how you can prevent it from happening in the future. It may be from feeling a sense of anxiety, agitation, or depression. Properly identify, and confront, your emotions instead of taking out your frustration on food. It may help you to write down what you feel, or engage in activities that will distract you.

Awareness is key when combatting emotional, or stress, eating. This is because a lot of people tend to ent more by simply not paying attention to what they put into their mouths. This causes all kinds of problems because often, the foods that people stress-eat are convenience foods that are very unhealthy. Eating without full awareness will lead to overeating, making poor food choices, as well as the inability to truly enjoy the food.

Whether you are working or lounging in the comfort of your own home, avoid having food in areas that are readily and easily accessible. Take those cookies out of your desk drawer and remove that bag of chips from the coffee table. Every time you feel urges and cravings, determine where they come from and then work to prevent them. Practice restraint instead of succumbing to temptation. You will find that after a while your willpower is going to greatly increase.

37 Avoid eating while watching TV or going to the movies.

Many people don't realize how much food they consume while they are focused on their favorite movie or TV series. Avoid having food nearby or, if you really need to snack, prepare something healthy like carrot sticks before becoming preoccupied with a movie. That way, when the snack is gone you will not have anything else in front of you to eat. Of course, you must avoid going back to refill your snack plate. Eating while watching TV is a very bad habit to get into because then every time you watch TV you will feel the need to have some form of food in front of you. Therefore, it is best to leave the food in the kitchen, away from the TV.

38 Teach yourself to control cravings.

One of the common downfalls of any diet programs is not the diet itself, but the individual's attitude towards food. You need to view food as a necessity instead of a pleasure. Eat smaller meals several times throughout the day so that you don't become over hungry from skipping a meal. This way you will not feel the urge to simply reach for the quick and easy junk food as a means to satisfy your hunger. Self-discipline is a very important trait you need to cultivate so you don't constantly cave in to temptation. Another great way to avoid caving in to your cravings is to remove all of the junk food from your house. If there isn't anything there, then you won't be able to mindlessly eat it.

39   Get support from family and friends.

If you are following a special diet, or a health regimen, let people who truly care about you know what you are into so they can understand and adjust accordingly. Often times, they will be a great help and will take extra care to assist you in your plan. Sometimes, they may even join in with you and begin to eat a healthy diet as well. A support group is also very important to help you stay motivated. It also serves to provide the affirmation and encouragement when you need it the most. The bottom line is that you cannot go it alone. Get out there and seek support, because the more people you have reminding and encouraging you, the more likely it is that you will succeed.

40   Beat temptations through distraction.

Every time you find it overly difficult to resist temptation, keep yourself busy so you don't have to dwell on the thought. Distraction is one of the best methods of removing something from your mind. If are tempted to eat that chocolate bar, then keep yourself busy with something so that you are not constantly thinking about the chocolate bar. Of course, the best thing to do would be to simply get rid of the chocolate bar. The point is that you need to stay strong and resist the temptation. Allowing yourself to be lured into indulging in one cookie will most likely lead to another one.

41 Keep a diary or journal.

Writing down your thoughts and feelings is a very powerful activity, as it helps put things in perspective. It is also a great form of stress relief. When you write things down, you are getting them off your chest, so to speak. Therefore, you are releasing all of that tension and giving your mind a break. Another great benefit of writing things down is that it frees up your memory. Now, instead of having to remember all of those things, you only have to remember where you wrote them down.

In addition, journaling is also an excellent way to track your progress if you are trying to lose weight and get in shape. It may also be very helpful if you are starting a new diet plan and making your own food. If you write down what you eat everyday, how you made it, and whether or not you liked it, then you will know exactly what to eat and what not to eat in the future.

42 Don't overlook the importance of emotional fitness.

Your emotional wellbeing is as important as your physical fitness. In fact, it is more important. You must work very hard to keep your mental state healthy. If you have an unstable mind and a rock solid body then you really can't do much, can you? It is always better to have your mind than anything else. Therefore, take good care of your mental wellbeing. If you feel the need to vent or talk to someone, seek the company of trusted friends or family. You can also consider taking therapy sessions or visiting with a group.

The point is that you need to do whatever you need to do in order to stay sane and mentally sharp. A positive emotional state is the driving force behind your desire to become a healthier you. If you let that dwindle, then you may find yourself sitting around, watching TV, and eating cupcakes because it helps you "feel" better. Don't let this be you.

43 Don't indulge too much on one thing.

Anything of excess can be a bad thing. Remember, everything in moderation. It is very important that you be smart with your choices, and keep your food intake to a minimum. Eat smaller meals and healthy snacks throughout the entire day instead of only eating large meals. This will help your metabolism and your emotional wellbeing. If you practice only eating to nourish and nurture the body then you will not become a glutton.

Of course, food is only one side of the pendulum. You need to make sure that you aren't overindulging in other areas of your life, such as work, school, or hobbies. Do everything in moderation and be sure to change it up every now and then. That way things will continue to be new and exciting rather than becoming old and boring.

44   Find a fitness buddy.

If you are a people person, it may be easier to stick to a health and fitness program if you have someone who can share your journey. It is also great to have someone to hang out with when you are working out. That way you guys can rotate with each other on the machines and push each other to do another set. You are hundreds of times more likely to work out longer, and do more, if you have a workout buddy pushing you than if you were to work out alone.

It is also more fun to engage in activities and try out healthy recipes with someone. If you guys are cooking, and something doesn't work out, then it becomes a great story and a memory. However, if you did it alone then you may become frustrated and discouraged. Basically, most things are easier, more memorable, and more fun when you are with people. Therefore, do yourself a huge favor and find someone to go through this with you.

45   Ride a bike to work.

If possible, you may want to consider riding a bicycle to work. It's a far healthier mode of transportation. Not only is it healthier, but also think of all the money you could save on vehicle expenses if you rode your bike more often. If you live within five miles of your destination then consider taking your bike. It won't take as long as you think. In addition, if you live near public transportation you could bike there and then use the transportation. Often times you can bring your bike on the bus and then ride it the rest of the way to your destination. It all depends on how motivated you are to do certain things. As always, before you embark upon any activity make sure you are prepared to do so. Have all the necessary safety equipment and emergency materials in case something goes wrong. After all, you definitely don't want to be late for work.

46   Be conscious with your food portions.

Even if you are eating healthy, but are eating too much, it defeats the purpose of diet and taking everything in moderation. Many people still gain weight by eating healthy. That is because they eat four or five large meals a day instead of using moderation and eating four or five smaller meals a day. When you eat, your meals should be proportioned correctly. A good guide is to eat a meal that is about the size of your hand flat with fingers together. Your snacks should be about the size of your fist if it was flat, not the whole 3D fist.

47   Increase fiber in your daily diet.

Fiber aids in weight loss and prevents constipation. It can also help avoid the build up of toxins in the body, which may lead to other health complications. It is a healthy food that you should begin to work into your diet.

Following a high-fiber diet can help effectively reduce the risks of heart diseases, colon cancer, diabetes, as well as diverticular diseases. It also works well in lowering the cholesterol levels. To increase fiber in the diet, here are some basic guidelines:

Increase consumption of grains and cereals – oat bran, wheat germ, whole-wheat flour products, and high-fiber cereals

Increase consumption of beans and legumes – kidney beans, legumes, and garbanzos
Fruits and veggies – fruits and vegetables, carrots, bananas

48   Enjoy after dinner walks.

If you have your family around, establish the routine of enjoying quiet walks around the neighborhood after a meal. Not only is it an excellent way to burn off some calories after a meal, it is also a great time for conversation. If you are by yourself, still get out there for a walk. Think of all the activity you may see, not to mention you will get to know your neighborhood very well.

According to studies, moderate intensity exercises, like brisk walking, can promote better weight loss. As a general rule, for you to shed of a single pound, you will need to burn about 3,500 calories. A half hour walk helps to burn off an estimated 150 calories. Contrary to popular belief, the act of walking after dinner will not cause muscle cramps. In fact, it will jump start your metabolism so your food will be burned faster than it would if you went to the couch.

49 Bake, steam, or grill instead of frying.

Deep fried dishes are high in cholesterol, so it's best to avoid them. If you really need to use cooking oil in your meals, opt for olive oil, as it is a far healthier alternative. Olive oil is high in essential fatty acids, or EFA's, which are good for your brain. One of the first things that you should do when you decide that you want to become fit and healthy is to get rid of all of the vegetable, canola, and other cheap oils in your house. In addition, get rid of that shortening, and Crisco as well. Extra virgin olive oil should be your only go-to for all your cooking needs.

50 Avoid eating at all you can eat buffets.

This should go without saying because if you go to an all you can eat buffet you will most likely over indulge in something. You generally don't want to put yourself in a position where it is difficult to resist temptation. That said, try to avoid going to buffets. In fact, try to avoid going out to eat all together. It will not only save you money, but will also be excellent for your health.

51 Only take enough food you can eat.

Avoid indulging in second and third helpings. Only place enough food on your plate that you are willing to consume, so you can avoid over-indulging. With that said, that doesn't mean you can load up your plate with two or three helpings so that you won't have to go back for more. No, it doesn't work like that. You need to only eat a moderate portion of food.

A great way to help you with this is to leave all the food on the stove instead of placing it on the table. If you dish up your food, and don't have it all in front of you, then you will be less likely to eat more of it. You will only consume the food available on the table and avoid excessive eating. If you plan to make large dishes to store, store it in containers and freeze it for your lunch or later meals. That way you will have some healthy and convenient fast food choices.

52   Start your meals with salads.

Before enjoying the main course, have a plate of green salad with some vegetables mixed in. Be careful with your choice dressing and the amount that you use, as some dressings are very bad for you. Eating a salad before your meal will help you feel fuller when you start the main course. It is also very good for you to eat so many greens at every meal.

By filling up your body with water-rich and fiber-rich food, you can effectively avoid overindulging on high-calorie meals. In fact, in a study conducted at Penn State, eating salads before a meal can reduce consumption of calories by as much as 12%.

53   Replace sugar with honey.

Consider using organic honey instead of sugar in your beverages and baked products as a healthier option. Honey is one of nature's greatest food products. It is something that will never spoil and will always be good for you. Honey helps heal your skin and has great medicinal properties. If you should use table sugar, opt for brown sugar as it contains fewer chemicals. Make sure that whatever sugar you use is pure cane sugar instead of sugar beet sugar.

Honey is a perfect alternative to regular sugar, since honey is generally sweeter than regular table sugar. This means you can use less honey than sugar. However, be extra careful when substituting sweeteners in recipes, since honey has its own distinct flavor, which can potentially ruin your baked goods.

54   Avoid skipping meals.

A lot of people seem to think that the best way to lose weight is to skip meals. This can have a detrimental effect, as it causes fluctuations in your blood sugar levels and can trigger excessive hunger, which can lead to overeating. Skipping a meal also puts your body in power saving mode so that it begins to store fat cells. Therefore, if you skip meals you are really defeating the purpose of your intention. Skipping meals slows your metabolism and is detrimental to weight loss and getting in shape. The best practice is to stick to eating small, frequent meals.

55 Trade baked goods with fresh fruits.

Pastries, cakes, and cookies are all high in carbohydrates and sugar, which can lead to weight gain. Carbs are simply bad for you. There is no other way to put it, and when you mix those bad for you carbs with bad for you sugar, you have a recipe for disaster. Therefore, try to avoid sweets as much as possible. If you need to eat something sweet, then have fruit instead. Fruits are loaded with sugar, and can often satisfy that same craving. However, if you are craving carbs, then try eating a half-cup of raw steel cut oats with milk or cream poured on top. It may seem strange at first, but eventually, this will be a wonderful little snack to help get you through a carb craving.

56 When eating out, choose the healthiest meals.

When you go out to eat there are many temptations and some of the pictures in the menu may seem to call your name. However, you must learn the art of choosing healthier meal options. Avoid ordering things because they look good. Order things because they sound good and look like they have a lot of healthy ingredients. It can also help if you share your meal with the people you are with. That way, you will avoid overeating. Of course, if you are by yourself then only eat half of your meal, and take the rest home for another time. There is no question about it, going out to eat when you are trying to stay healthy is a hard thing to do. Therefore, it is best simply to avoid going out to eat. You will not only save money, but you will also avoid the temptations of unhealthy foods.

57   Avoid using condiments.

Some condiments are generally bad for the health, so try to avoid using them as much as possible. While condiments are known to add more flavor and aroma to food, there are those that come fully loaded with sugar and preservatives, which pose serious health risks. Here are some pointers on what you can use and what to avoid:

Enjoy the following condiments:

- Mustard
- Hot sauce
- Vinegars
- Cream cheese
- Worcestershire sauce
- Horseradish
- Pesto
- Soy sauce
- Sour cream

Avoid the following condiments:

- Barbecue sauce
- Maple syrup (unless it is natural)
- Teriyaki sauce
- Ketchup
- Cocktail sauce

- Regular jellies and jams

58 When traveling, check out gym facilities.

Traveling out of town, or out of the country, should not disrupt your regular exercise regimen. Don't let traveling become an excuse to stop you from working out. It will serve to break the great habit that you worked so hard to develop. Often times, when you get home you will continue that break from working out, and your habit will die off. Therefore, when you are traveling, check out available facilities, and include exercise in your itinerary. You can also bring along a few simple gym items like a jump rope or an elastic band if you want to exercise in the comfort of your hotel room. A workout DVD would also be another excellent choice.

59 Do your research on local restaurants that offer healthy alternatives.

When being in an unfamiliar place, it can be all too easy to eat what is convenient and readily available. To help you stick to your diet, check out healthy options within the area. You can always ask the front desk for assistance. The key is that you need to be willing and determined to seek out the healthy food options. If you are lazy, and choose to eat at the restaurant within your hotel, then your diet plan has gone straight out the window. You need to maintain that self-discipline and motivation. Don't let travel ruin everything you have built. Stay strong and find the healthy options. You may even find that it is an adventure to find those healthy options instead of lazily going wherever is convenient.

60 Bring your lunch.

Instead of grabbing a quick bite at the cafeteria, or a nearby fast food chain, bring along your lunch. Most workplaces have a break room with a refrigerator and microwave so there should be no excuse. If your workplace doesn't have these options then bring your lunch in a cooler. This will give you better control on what types of foods you eat and how much you consume. You need to make the choice, and be willing to put in the effort, to bring your own lunch everyday. It really isn't that difficult. All you need to do is make extra when you cook your evening meals and store the leftovers in the frig, or freezer, for your future lunches.

61 Trade your recliner with an exercise ball.

The growing trend among modern offices today is the use of exercise balls in place of ordinary office chairs. This is a perfect option for people whose work requires them to spend long hours behind a desk. Exercise balls will require you to maintain proper posture and use muscles for balance. It is a good passive workout for desk-bound employees. Another great advantage is that exercise balls are far less expensive than regular office chairs. Therefore, don't be afraid to be the only one with a ball. Chances are, others will follow your lead. Of course, make sure to clear it with your employer first.

62 Use your break time wisely.

Instead of taking a nap or chatting with your colleagues, maximize your break time by going out for a short walk. It can be a good idea to bring along some comfy shoes that you can use, in case your work shoes are not ideal for walking. If you miss the social interaction, then invite a co-worker to walk around with you. Start small by asking them if they want to walk a little bit. Then gradually increase the distance. Before you know it, the two of you will be climbing stairs on your breaks!

63 Conduct a meeting on the go.

Instead of staying cooped up in the conference room, maximize time by conducting your meeting outdoors, or while walking towards another location. This will not only save you time, it presents a perfect excuse to stretch your legs and exercise. Of course, the other people in your meeting will have to be willing to walk with you. Unless it is a phone meeting that you can do on the go. As always, make sure you are prepared for the meeting. You don't want to get away from your desk and then all of a sudden need a file that is on your computer. You need to be smart about what you do so that your work is not affected.

64   Invest in a pedometer.

This is a small device that you can wear to automatically count the number of steps you take in a day. It will help you keep track of the miles that you walk each day. In addition, it will serve as a reminder, and guide, for you throughout the day. Some cell phones and watches have this function built into the app database, along with many other fitness tools. Knowing the number of steps you take in a day can be a great tool that you can use to help you reach your fitness objectives even while at the office, or while running some errands.

65   Learn to modify.

Every so often you may find yourself in situations where it is difficult to stick to your fitness routine. The trick here is to learn to adjust to those situations. You need to be flexible and adaptable. If you don't have dumbbells around, you can use canned goods or water bottles as alternative options. Learn to make use of available resources and be creative. You cannot afford to let your health suffer. If you take a break from your daily workout and good eating routines then it will be very hard to get back into it. You will lose your momentum. Essentially, you are stopping in the middle of the hill and then continuing your climb. Don't do it.

66 Take vacations from work, not from good health.

Traveling and enjoying a holiday vacation should not be an excuse to indulge in foods that are generally bad for your health. Simply because all of the foods are there and readily available doesn't mean they are all there for you. Sure it is okay to have a piece of pie or some cookies on the holidays, but be careful not to eat them constantly throughout the holidays. In addition, all that great food is excellent, and you will definitely be tempted to over eat. Remember, there will be leftovers and you can enjoy them later on. Don't get caught up in the moment and allow your health routine to diminish.

67 Learn to express your feelings.

Keeping your emotions bottled up will contribute to stress, and increase the risk of health related problems such as heart attacks, substance abuse, depression, and anxiety. Therefore, don't keep things in. Let them out, and either write them down or talk to someone. When you begin to feel agitated, frustrated, or some other negative emotion, take a break. Then think about it and determine the triggers for those feelings. Ask yourself if that was a proper reaction to the trigger. Everything is a matter of perspective, perhaps next time you can react differently. Over time, you can train yourself to avoid all negative emotions and learn to embrace positivity in your words, actions, and thoughts.

68   Maintain a positive attitude.

Life will not always go your way so get used to that. Instead of wallowing in failures and disappointments, learn to brush it off and move forward. You need to keep a positive attitude and make the best of every situation. Spending your time and energy whining, complaining, or pouting will get you nowhere. It will only serve to drain your emotional state and decrease your mentality. Therefore, whether it is a failed relationship, a lost opportunity, or an unsavory situation, choose to see the positive side of things and maintain a happy disposition. This will help you channel your energies to the right direction and rise up to the challenges ahead instead of falling beneath them.

69   Try meditation.

Meditation is a very great thing for your mind and body. It involves the control of breathing patterns and enhancing focus. This will help you clear away mental cobwebs and maintain better perspective on situations. By learning the right breathing patterns, you will be able to provide your brain the right oxygen supply to clear away mental disturbances. Don't be afraid to go to a class, or sign up for group sessions. In addition, you can also get some DVD's and do them at home. Sometimes meditation is included in some great exercise routines, like yoga, so you can get your workout in as well as clear your mind.

70   Reinforce your faith.

Everybody needs something to believe in. Even atheists believe in something. Humans long to believe that there are things that are beyond their control. People need the security that someone is there watching out for them. Therefore, develop and seek spiritual enlightenment and focus beyond material wealth. This will help you attain lasting happiness and satisfaction, which are difficult to derive from material possessions. By reinforcing your faith, you can also promote better overall health and wellbeing. The act of going to church, or other religious functions, can also be a great way to meet friends that will be very supportive and helpful to you.

71   Stay young at heart.

Age is only in the mind. Yes, your body will begin to decay, as you get older, but don't let that get you down. You are as young, or as old, as you choose to be. So be careful not to take things too seriously and learn to enjoy life a little. Remember, everything in moderation. Have a balance and know when to be serious and when to loosen up and have fun. Take the time to enjoy life's simple pleasures, and remember that laughter is the best anti-aging solution that is available for free. It can also help boost the immune system. Therefore, get out there and enjoy yourself once in a while.

72   Stay in touch with friends.

Despite the popularity of online social networking sites, it should not replace your personal interactions with the people around you. Indulge in regular conversations and preserve real life social networks by joining groups. Stay in touch with friends, and plan activities together. The computer is a great way to keep in touch, but don't let it become your only method of interaction. You need to get out in the world and do things with friends. This will keep you active, which will do wonders for your health and wellbeing.

73   Perform regular stretching exercises.

Stretching is the best way to work out a few kinks and aches from staying in a position for far too long, like working on a computer. If you have a job where you sit for extended periods of time then make a point to get up and walk around every so often. In addition, stand up and stretch every now and then. Make an effort to find some yoga classes, or buy a DVD that you can do at home. Stretching increases blood flow, circulation, and jumpstarts the body. It is something that you should do every morning, if possible. The health benefits are too numerous to count. Therefore, make stretching a part of your regular day. It is something that is fast, simple, easy, and very effective.

74   Keep talking.

According to research, talking at least ten minutes a day, to another person, can promote better brain function and enhance memory. It is also good for your vocabulary and social skills. Talking with people can serve to boost your brainpower, and being social has been linked to a longer lifespan. Talking allows you a form of release. You feel like your voice was heard and that provides a form of satisfaction, which is very important for your mental health. Therefore, make an effort to talk to someone everyday.

75   Stop smoking.

One can't stress enough the risks and ill effects of smoking. It limits the oxygen supply to the body, and leads to a host of health complications including shortened life expectancy rate. It has also been found that smoking can indirectly contribute to back pain. In addition, smoking has adverse effects on people around you. Second-hand smokers have been known to suffer significantly increased risks of health complications that can even lead to death. Think of the money that you pour into smoking every month. If you are a smoker and you want to become healthy then you need to quit. Health and smoking do not go together at all.

76   Aim high.

Set your weight and health goals, and then break them into smaller milestones. This will keep you motivated and focused on achieving your goals. Write each one down and place them in places that are readily available to you. That way you can easily see them everyday and they will serve as a constant reminder and motivate you to achieve them. Post a copy on your refrigerator, work desk, and laptop. The thing to remember is to set very high goals. Then break them down and work on them one step at a time. That way, as you accomplish each step, you will be reinforced with satisfaction. This will motivate you to keep working toward your next goal.

77   Keep yourself updated.

Conduct regular research, and stay updated on the latest health discoveries. The Internet provides many great resources on new exercise routines, new health spas in your area, and any other health and fitness-related interests. You need to make the effort to continue learning. Finding out, and trying, new things will help you to stay motivated. After all, if you find a new recipe on Pinterest and try it out, you will be motivated to look for more. This will help prevent you from growing tired of eating the same foods all the time. There are so many possibilities out there, and your health routine can change daily if you want it to.

78   Know your body.

Determine what the factors are that trigger weight gain for you. Also, learn the best nutrition for your specific body type. This will help you in making day-to-day decisions. Everyone's body is different, and will require different weight loss and nutrition approaches. Know how different foods, and exercise routines, affect you, and find those that are most effective in helping you achieve your goals. Take the time to study different types and expand your knowledge. That way, if someone has a question, you may be able to help him or her through your experience. This will not only help them stay motivated, but it will help you. If you have someone that you are mentoring, then you will be motivated to be a good role model for him or her.

79   Grill it up.

When the weather permits, use your outdoor grill to cook your food. Grilling can be an excellent alternative to traditional cooking, and it will help keep your house cool on those hot summer days. There are many arguments about whether or not grilling is healthy. However, if you grill healthy foods then it really doesn't matter. There is nothing wrong with grilling as long as you don't load up your food with sauces and other marinades. Therefore, don't be afraid to start grilling your food.

80   Treat your brain like any other muscle.

Much like any other muscle in the body, your brain also needs regular exercise. Enjoy board games, crossword puzzles, and any other activity that presents a mental challenge. The more you use your brain the better it will become. You need to work it out and engage in activities where you think and are challenged. Your brain needs to solve problems and be stressed in small amounts. Learning presents the brain with a good form of stress that will keep your mind sharp and active. Your mind is one thing that you don't want to lose. Therefore, make the effort to keep it.

81   Get nutty.

Nuts are a very healthy snack option that can effectively stave off food cravings. They are high in fats, proteins, and good carbohydrates. However, make sure to choose the unsalted and roasted varieties, as they are known to be free from sugars and sodium. Basically, you want to get nuts that are pure. That means that it is the nut only. Consuming nuts that are caked in sugar, wasabi sauce, honey, or any other type of glaze defeats the purpose. You need to eat whole foods, and that means eating nuts that are lightly salted or dry roasted. When choosing nuts, opt for the healthy nuts like almonds, walnuts, pecans, et cetera. Try to stay away from peanuts, as these really aren't that great for you.

82   Stay protected.

The sun is a very powerful source of cosmic rays. These rays can be damaging to your overall health and wellbeing. Therefore, you must take action to shield yourself from them if you want to stay healthy. Remember to apply sunblock, especially when you are spending a significant amount of time outside and have skin exposed. The sun can damage your skin and can cause wrinkles. This will make you look older and have premature aging. In addition, chronic sunburn can also cause cancer and lots of problems down the road.

83   Mind your posture.

Stand up straight. Everyone has heard that over and over when they were growing up. Unfortunately, many people never headed that advice. Good posture will help you in more ways than you can imagine. If you stand up straight, you will look taller, more intelligent, and in better shape than people who don't stand up straight. Good posture helps to protect your back from unnecessary damage. In addition, maintaining proper posture can enhance mental focus and promote better blood circulation.

84   Avoid processed food products.

Always choose fresh, whole foods as much as possible. Anything else is going to be hazardous to your health. In general, foods that are packaged in boxes, bags, and cans have been altered and are highly processed. Although they are convenient, the packaging process makes them devoid of essential nutrients and laden with preservatives and chemicals. That means that these foods only serve to fill you up and then add toxins to your body. This causes your body to work harder to remove those toxins. It also damages the systems in your body. Therefore, try to avoid all of the premade convenience foods, and take the time to make your own food from real whole foods.

85 Always carry a water bottle wherever you go.

This is one of the most practical ways you can stay fit and hydrated all throughout the day. Water is something that many people don't pay enough attention to. It is possibly the most important ailment prevention in history. Water can help you stay very healthy, and will prevent so many problems that you really must drink plenty of it. Water can effectively reduce hunger cravings, prevent you from overeating, prevent irritability, headaches, cramps, and promote proper body functioning.

Make it a goal to drink a gallon of water per day. Of course, you probably won't hit that mark, but in doing so you will definitely get enough water. Get yourself a water bottle that has the ounces written on the side. A 32-ounce would be perfect, then you can shoot for drinking four of them per day. That would be plenty of water. Add that to the coffee, juice, milk, and other liquids you consume, and you will be perfectly hydrated.

86 Get plenty of fresh air.

Revitalize your body by inhaling fresh air. Make a point to spend an hour or so outside everyday. While you are out there, take a few deep breaths every now and then. This will help fill your lungs with some good fresh air. Enclosed workspaces can reduce natural airflow, which makes you more susceptible to diseases.

Prevent that by opening windows, and limiting your time inside. Fresh air also helps you sleep better. When you spend long portions of time outside, your body will feel more natural and will feel like it worked all day long. As a result, it will sleep better because it believes it is more tired. Try it out. Spend a day outside and see how you sleep.

87   Take advantage of natural sunlight.

Early morning sunlight can help boost your immune system and has been known to combat depression. Therefore, make an effort to get outside and spend some time in the sun. Sunlight is something that is excellent for your emotional health. After all, how many people do you know that have a light they turn on for a certain time during the day to improve their mood? Seasonal Affective Disorder is becoming a very popular problem because people are spending so much time indoors. Prevent this from happening to you by getting out in the sun for an hour or so a day. Remember to protect your skin though.

88   Take the stairs.

Instead of using the elevator, use the opportunity for a quick workout by taking the stairs. This will not only be good for your daily step count, but will also help to keep you in shape. Often times, taking the stairs may be a little quicker than waiting around for the elevator, especially if you only need to travel a few floors. In addition, when you are on an escalator, instead of standing there and waiting for it to bring you to the top. Take the opportunity to walk up and get there twice as fast! You must always be thinking about how you can work a little exercise into your daily routine.

89   For women, visit gynecologist regularly.

Females eighteen and above should undergo an annual physical examination that includes a Pap Smear test. In addition, those in their forty's should have mammograms along with regular breast self-examination to ensure early detection. Unfortunately, breast cancer is a very popular thing. Therefore, you must pay attention and stay on top of your health maintenance so that cancer can be avoided. Breasts are a highly coveted body part in this world; do you want to lose yours?

90   Walk and stretch during road travel.

When taking road trips, make sure to take frequent stops so you have a chance to walk around the vicinity and stretch the muscles. This will not only protect your back and help you burn calories, stretching can also help you stay more alert on the road when driving. Regular stops will help you feel better upon reaching your destination. It will also provide you with the opportunity to see more along your journey. Think of all the interesting places that you drive through, all of the cool little stores, towns, and shops, that you would be able to see if you stopped. Go ahead and leave a little earlier so that you can take your time getting to your destination and stop along the way.

91   Visit your dentist regularly.

Good oral hygiene is also an important part of overall health and wellness. You need to make sure that you are brushing your teeth a minimum of twice a day. In addition, flossing once per day is essential. Depending on your personal oral health, it may also be a great idea to use mouthwash. Of course, you also need to visit your dentist at least once a year. The current recommendation is that you go twice a year for a cleaning. However, this can be expensive. Therefore, check with your insurance. Some companies offer one or two free cleanings a year as a preventative measure. If this isn't an option for you, then take a look at some local universities. Often times they will perform dental work for a tenth of the regular cost.

92   Workout with kids.

Spend the weekend playing with kids. This is the perfect opportunity to bond and spend leisure time away from the daily stresses of grown up life. Plan a park, or beach, outing or even a trip to the zoo. Keeping up with active toddlers and preschoolers can turn out to be a fun exercise for you. Not only will it help keep you active, but it will also help you stay young. In addition, you may enjoy some of those childhood activities. Now you have the perfect opportunity to play those games, as an adult, and having it appear normal.

93   Substitute emails for walks.

When working in an office, instead of emailing your colleague, grab this opportunity to walk over and discuss things personally. This will not only speed up the communication process, it also provides you with the opportunity to stretch and walk. In addition, you will get out of your chair and have a change of scenery. This may help you be more productive when you get back to your desk. However, make sure that you are only going over there to ask about something that is important and work related. You shouldn't be hindering their productivity, or the productivity of others, by constantly walking to different co-workers and asking them pointless questions.

94   Warm up before exercise.

Launching your body into an intense physical exercise with cold muscles can increase the risks of injuries. In fact, a lot of sports-related injuries can be prevented through proper stretching and warm-ups. Whether it's a high impact sport like basketball, or a grueling game of golf, never undermine the importance of properly warming up the muscles to prevent strains and sprains, as well as cramps.

However, the practice of warming up may be overrated. After all, do you ever see a lion warm up before taking down a gazelle? No. Therefore, the best practice is to know your body. Some people are more prone to injuries than others. So if you only need five minutes to warm up and are good, then go with it. If someone else needs a half hour, then give him or her a half hour. Know your body.

95   Take a stand.

You will be surprised to know that standing can burn up to 34 more calories compared to sitting down. In addition, people who stand more often than they sit can live up to six years longer. So you can ditch the standard work desk and get one that features vertical adjustments. Of course, this will have to be approved by your employer. However, many companies now make attachments that you can place on top of your regular desk. The attachment provides a lift that comes up so that you can now stand at your desk. Then when you need to sit, simply lower the lift back down to your regular desktop height. Try to do as many things as you can while standing. For example, when answering phones, stand up and walk around, so you can burn calories at the same time.

96   Park farther.

Instead of fighting over who gets the prime spot in the parking lot, choose to park farther away, preferably a full block from the office. This will give you the opportunity to walk and stretch on a daily basis. It will also help ensure that you remember to get everything out of your car. If you know you are parking farther away, you will be less likely to run to your car because you forgot something. In addition, it may also help keep your car free of those annoying door dings. If you park where no one else wants to park then you will have less chance of some fool banging into your car.

97 Use chicken breast and take off the skin.

Chicken is such a great meat. It is so versatile, that you can use it in almost any type of meal. Chicken is also very healthy for you because it is a lean protein that is metabolized very quickly. When cooking, work with breast portions, as they contain the most amount of white meat, which is healthier than the dark meat. Make sure to remove the skin because that is high in fat and cholesterol. Some people really enjoy the skin, and if that is you then don't worry about eating it. As long as you aren't eating it three times a day then you will be fine. Basically, if you are eating chicken instead of other meats, especially pork, then you are already a leg up on being healthy. Make sure that you don't drown it in sauces, as they can contain so many preservative and a lot of sugar.

98 Learn to decipher food labels.

This is one skill that will prove handy when making smarter food choices. Get used to reading the ingredient labels on anything that you eat. You must know what you are eating. If there is something that you don't know what it is, then look it up. Generally, if you don't know what it is, or can't say it, then you really shouldn't be eating it. However, an even easier way to determine whether or not you should eat something is to skip everything with an ingredient list.

Of course some things, like peanut butter, have an ingredient list and are still okay. But make sure that the list is only peanuts and salt. You don't want to be eating peanut butter with sugar and added preservatives. Generally, if you stick to whole foods with no ingredients list, and foods with very short ingredient lists, then you will be perfectly fine.

99   Just chew it.

If you are dealing with a sweet tooth, try substituting your usual dessert with gum. This will keep your mouth busy and provide the distraction you need to keep your mind off dessert. However, be careful which gum you choose. Some people may have sensitivities to the different preservatives in gum. You most likely know what type of gum you enjoy chewing so don't worry about it. In fact, even regular sugared gum isn't worth fretting over unless you are chewing five pieces, or more, a day.

100 Always choose to plan ahead.

It can be significantly easier to stick to eating regimen if you plan ahead. Prepare the menu for the following week so you don't have to spend extra time racking your brain on what to cook and how to prepare your food. Having a weekly menu can also effectively discourage the need to order food delivery and take-out. It will also make your grocery shopping go much faster and easier. If you know what you need, and exactly what you are going to cook, then you can make a list and stick to it. This will help save you money because you aren't purchasing additional items that you don't need.

101 Keep moving forward.

People tend to be more motivated when they have a goal in mind. You need to have a purpose or you will never succeed. In general, people only do things when there is something in it for them, when there is something to look forward to. So the lesson here is to always have a goal, and not only with your health and fitness, but your overall wellbeing.

Conclusion

Hopefully, you have learned some valuable information and these tips will help you in your goal to become a healthier you. By keeping a healthy body and eating right, you will open yourself up to a great new world of opportunities. As the saying goes, if you want to be successful, you have to act, feel, and look every bit as successful as you want to be. These days, financial status is not the only yardstick used to measure success. The appearance of a healthy and fit body is also critically important in wielding respect and commanding authority.

Incorporate all these tips, tricks, and pointers into your lifestyle. While it may take a while to adjust and transition into a number of changes, investing in good health will never be too expensive. In addition, you may want to take a look at some of the articles and other resources listed on www.spencercoffman.com. There are a wide variety of tools and ideas there that will help you in your endeavor to become a healthier you.

Good Luck!

~Spencer Coffman

Appendix A:

Checklist

You've read the book, A Healthier You by Spencer Coffman, now it's time to start putting those healthy living tips into action. It's time to start cracking down and being determined to live a healthier lifestyle so you can start feeling better, having more energy, and truly become a healthier you!

To do that, you're going to need to remember everything you've learned and make it a reality in your life. That's where the A Healthier You Checklist will come in handy. Work through this selection, and you should be a lot closer to achieving the kind of lifestyle you want and finally achieving the type of body that you deserve. You'll start to look and feel better; you'll have more self-confidence, and finally be able to wear anything you like without feeling self-conscious.

A HEALTHIER YOU!

In the full book, we discussed 101 powerful tips that you can use to become a fitter, healthier, you. You learned, in detail, how to make those suggestions a reality. This checklist will serve as sort of an outline for the book so that you will be able to keep all of these tips and ideas right at your fingertips.

Of course, this is only a checklist. You'll still need to read through the full book if you truly desire to live a healthier life and become the person you have always dreamed of being. Anyway, here is the A Healthier You Checklist.

Stay Active

Staying active is the number one way to stay healthy. If you are active, your body learns to be active. It's simple science – a body in motion stays in motion, whereas a body at rest tends to stay at rest. Be a body in motion.

- Exercise Your Mind And Body

- Trade Chairs For Exercise Balls

- Find Gyms When Traveling

- Park Further Away

- Take The Stairs

- Go For Walks

Strive To Eat Right

The foods you eat will directly impact your health. You need to make sure you are eating regularly and consistently. Your body needs to be able to count on your food intake so that it can do its job providing you with energy and health.

- Eat Your Breakfast

- Have 5 to 6 Meals A Day

- Go Organic

- Control Your Cravings

- Avoid Skipping Meals

- Watch The Snacks

Mind Your Fluid Intake

Hydration is probably the most important aspect of health. After all, without water you will not last long. Therefore, make sure to stay hydrated with water. Be careful of the other beverages because they are loaded with additives. Drink water and lots of it.

- Stay Hydrated

- Drink Green Tea

- Moderate Your Alcohol

- Limit The Caffeine

Boost Your Immune System

Your immune system is your defense against poor health. Therefore, you need to make sure you have a strong immune system so your body will be able to fight off any attacks to your health.

- Get Enough Sleep

- Wash Your Hands

- Take Fish Oil

- Take Vitamins

- Get Health Checkups

- Visit Your Dentist

Maintain Relationships

Relationships are important for your mental health and wellbeing. Humans are social creatures. Use this to your advantage by finding and nurturing good, positive, relationships with people and getting rid of bad, negative, relationships.

- Find A Fitness Buddy

- Avoid Negative People

- Bask In Love

- Get Support From Others

- Stay In Touch With Friends

Make Healthy Choices

The foundation of your health lies in your ability to make healthy choices. You need to actively choose things that are going to be good for you. If you don't, then you'll follow ease and convenience, which are notoriously bad for your health.

- Ditch The Chips

- Watch Your Portions

- Select Healthy Food From The Menu

- Avoid All You Can Eat

- Be Careful Of Stress Eating

Your Spiritual Self

Mental health is exactly as important as physical health. Your brain is a muscle and you need to make sure that you are working it as well. Take the time and effort to make sure your mind is healthy, because after all, your mind controls your body.

- Learn Relaxation Techniques

- Express Your Feelings

- Maintain A Positive Attitude

- Try Meditation

- Reinforce Your Faith

- Stay Young At Heart

That's it! Use this checklist to refresh your memory on what you read in A Healthier You. Of course, there are many more great tips in the book. In addition, all of the tips are explained in detail, rather than simply listed. Therefore, if you haven't read it yet, I strongly encourage you to do so. That is, if you have a desire to become A Healthier You!

Spencer Coffman
SpencerCoffman.com

Appendix B:

Resource Cheat Sheet

Hopefully, by now you've read the book A Healthier You By Spencer Coffman. If so, you know what you can do to start living a healthier and energetic life. Your life has a way of always being busy, which means you opt for convenience foods rather than healthy foods. In addition, you may not exercise as much as you like or always follow healthy habits. Unfortunately, this isn't good for you and it causes you to feel tired and sluggish. Fortunately, A Healthier You provided you with some great tips to stay healthy even with your busy lifestyle.

Therefore, make an effort to incorporate what you learned in the book and maintain a healthy lifestyle. Of course, it is easier said than done, but nothing good comes easy. If you want to live a healthier and fitter life then you need to make some changes. Don't worry though; the A Healthier You Resource Cheat Sheet will help you stay on top of your health so you can become a fitter, healthier you!

Resources

Superfood Health Chart

http://spencercoffman.com/superfood-health-chart/

This is a great list of all kinds of foods that are amazing for your body. They are known as "Super Foods" which means they provide so many great nutrients that you should try to incorporate them into your diet.

The Diet Quiz

http://www.weightlossjoy.com/the-diet-quiz/

Weight Loss Joy presents... The Diet Quiz! Now you are only a few questions away from finding your ideal diet plan. You must be very honest with yourself so that you will get some results that you can use. Go ahead and give it a try!

Choosing The Right Diet

http://www.mayoclinic.org/healthy-lifestyle/weight-loss/in-depth/weight-loss/art-20048466

Mayo Clinic is an authority figure when it comes to health. In this great article, they walk you through everything you need to know so that you can select the diet that is right for you.

Choosing The Right Workout For You

http://www.fitnessmagazine.com/workout/tips/best-workout-for-you/

Fitness Magazine has a lot of great articles and resources in the health niche. Here is a pretty good resource to use when deciding what you are going to do to stay in shape.

Drink More Water!

http://spencercoffman.com/drink-more-water/

Perhaps the most important thing when it comes to your health is making sure you drink plenty of water. Water is probably the best thing for your body and you need to make sure you get enough. Take a look at this great article for more reasons why you need to drink more water!

Tools

iPhone Health App

https://www.apple.com/ios/health/

This is an amazing app that you can use to track many of your fitness goals. In addition, it is also a platform. This means it allows other apps to work, and communicate, with it. Definitely take the time to learn how to use this app.

Health Apps For Droid Users

http://www.androidauthority.com/best-health-apps-for-android-668268/

If you don't have an iPhone, then you should still find an app that can help you out. Androids have a number of apps that you can use. Go ahead and select one from the list and put it into action.

How To Check Your Recovery Rate

http://spencercoffman.com/recovery-rate/

It's important to know how quickly you recover after working out. There are several methods of checking your recovery rate. Go ahead and choose the one that's right for you!

Heart Rate Monitor

http://amzn.to/2ewbGLe

Staying on top of your heart rate is very important if you are trying to stay fit and healthy. You can do this with a heart rate monitor and there are several options available.

Books

A Healthier You by Spencer Coffman

http://spencercoffman.com/a-healthier-you/

If you haven't already read it, here's your chance. This book will show you 101 powerful tips to live a healthier lifestyle.

The Four-Hour Body by Tim Ferris
http://amzn.to/2pR9Yt5

Once again Tim Ferris has another great resource for you. This book is filled with all kinds of information to help you get the body you want.

The Whole 30 by Melissa Hartwig
http://amzn.to/2ppAc4u

Here is a great guide that you can use to get your health in order in only 30 days. It is a complete 30-day guide to achieve optimal health.

How Not To Die by Michael Greger
http://amzn.to/2qxW5MF

The title of this book should be enough in and of itself to get you to read it. However, in case it isn't, this book is all about the foods out there that can prevent and reverse disease. Check it out!

Your Body's Many Cries For Water by F. Batmanghelidj
http://amzn.to/2qrBDxF

It's no secret. Your body needs water. This book

details decades of research detailing how water can cure almost any ailment. At any rate, even if you don't read the book, start drinking more water!

Of course, there are many more great resources out there. However, the A Healthier You book, the Checklist, the Mind Map, and this Resource Cheat Sheet should be more than enough to get you started. Stick with it, and you'll be a fitter, healthier you in no time!

SpencerCoffman.com

Appendix C:

Mind Map

Here is the list version of the A Healthier You Mind Map. The flow chart is located online at SpencerCoffman. com. Go ahead and check it out so you can use it to help you with your fitness goals.

Stay Active

Exercise Your Mind And Body

Trade Chairs For Exercise Balls

Find Gyms When Traveling

Park Further Away

A HEALTHIER YOU!

Take The Stairs

Go For Walks

Strive To Eat Right

Eat Your Breakfast

Have 5 to 6 Meals A Day

Go Organic

Control Your Cravings

Avoid Skipping Meals

Watch The Snacks

Mind Your Fluid Intake

Stay Hydrated

Drink Green Tea

Moderate Your Alcohol

Limit The Caffeine

Boost Your Immune System

Get Enough Sleep

Mind Map

Wash Your Hands

Take Fish Oil

Take Vitamins

Get Health Checkups

Visit Your Dentist

Maintain Relationships

Find A Fitness Buddy

Avoid Negative People

Bask In Love

Get Support From Others

Stay In Touch With Friends

Make Healthy Choices

Ditch The Chips

Watch Your Portions

Select Healthy Food From The Menu

Avoid All You Can Eat

Be Careful Of Stress Eating

Your Spiritual Self

Learn Relaxation Techniques

Express Your Feelings

Maintain A Positive Attitude

Try Meditation

Reinforce Your Faith

Stay Young At Heart

Created by Spencer Coffman
SpencerCoffman.com

Mind Map

A HEALTHIER YOU!

About The Author

Having gone through several health trials of his own, a few of which were life threatening, Spencer Coffman knows the importance of living a healthy lifestyle and has made it his way of life. Now you can too! Read A Healthier You to find out how to live healthy the easy way. To read more about Spencer, visit his website spencercoffman.com

A HEALTHIER YOU!

About The Author